THE GALLBLADDER HEALTH FOR BEGINNERS

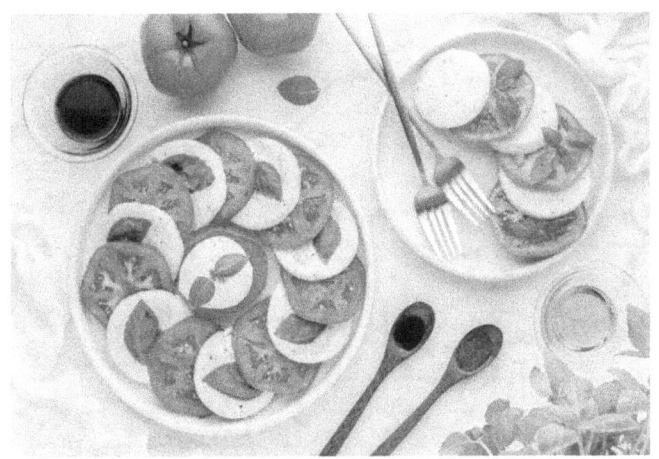

DR. JESSICA SMITH

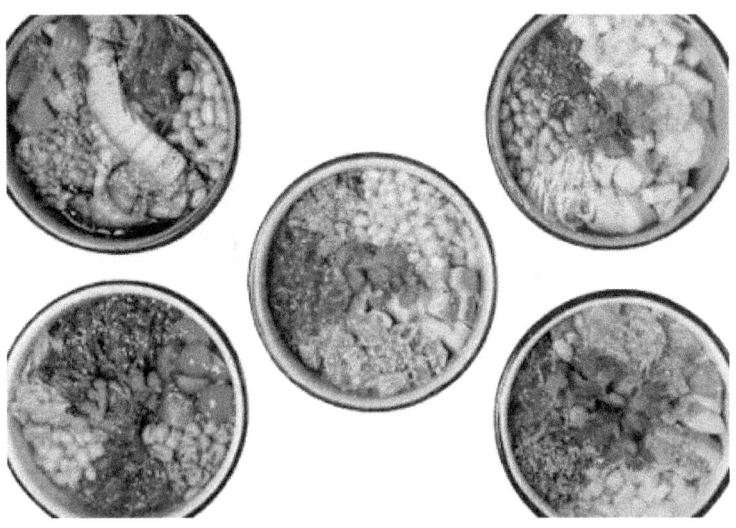

TABLE OF CONTENTS

CHAPTER ONE

How to Use this Cookbook

Stay Hydrated:

Ensure you drink an adequate amount of water daily. Hydration helps in maintaining the flow of bile, a crucial digestive fluid produced by the liver and stored in the gallbladder.

Incorporate Healthy Fats:

Choose sources of healthy fats such as avocados, olive oil, and fatty fish. These fats support the gallbladder's ability to release bile, aiding in the digestion of fats.

Eat Fiber-Rich Foods:

Include plenty of fiber in your diet through fruits, vegetables, and whole grains. Fiber helps regulate digestion and can prevent the formation of gallstones.

Limit Processed Foods:

Reduce the intake of processed and fried foods, as they can contribute to inflammation and may strain the gallbladder.

Control Portion Sizes:

Be mindful of portion sizes to prevent overeating, which can put extra stress on the gallbladder. Eating smaller, more frequent meals throughout the day may be beneficial.

Choose Lean Proteins:

Opt for lean protein sources like poultry, fish, and legumes. Lean proteins are easier for the body to digest, putting less strain on the gallbladder.

Maintain a Healthy Weight:

Aim for a healthy weight through a balanced diet and regular exercise. Excess body weight is a risk factor for gallstones and gallbladder issues.

Avoid Rapid Weight Loss:

If considering weight loss, do so gradually and through a well-balanced approach. Rapid weight loss can increase the risk of gallstones.

Include Herbal Support:

Some herbs like peppermint, turmeric, and dandelion may have positive effects on gallbladder function.

Consult with a healthcare professional before incorporating herbal supplements.

Listen to Your Body:

Pay attention to how your body responds to different foods. If you notice discomfort or digestive issues, consider keeping a food journal to identify potential triggers and seek guidance from a healthcare professional.

Understanding Gall Bladder Health for Beginners

Understanding gallbladder health is crucial for beginners embarking on a journey toward digestive well-being.

The gallbladder, a small organ beneath the liver, plays a vital role in the digestive system. Its primary function is to store bile, a fluid produced by the liver that aids in the digestion of fats.

For beginners, fostering gallbladder health involves making mindful dietary choices and adopting lifestyle practices that support optimal function.

Key elements of gallbladder health include maintaining a well-hydrated state, incorporating healthy fats into the diet, and embracing fiber-rich foods to regulate digestion. Beginners should strive to limit processed and fried foods, as these can contribute to inflammation and gallbladder strain.

Controlling portion sizes and choosing lean proteins also alleviates stress on the gallbladder, promoting smoother digestion.

Crucially, understanding gallbladder health involves recognizing the impact of weight on its function.

Maintaining a healthy weight through balanced nutrition and regular exercise is essential, as excess weight is a risk factor for gallstone formation.

Beginners should approach weight loss gradually, avoiding rapid changes that may increase the likelihood of gallbladder issues.

In essence, beginners in gallbladder health should listen to their bodies, be mindful of dietary choices, and consult healthcare professionals for personalized guidance.

This foundational understanding sets the stage for a proactive approach to digestive health, fostering a balanced and harmonious relationship with the gallbladder.

Principles of Gall Bladder Health for Beginners

Principles of gallbladder health for beginners center on fostering optimal digestion and minimizing the risk of gallbladder-related issues. Key principles include:

Balanced Diet:

Embrace a well-balanced diet rich in fruits, vegetables, whole grains, and lean proteins. This provides essential nutrients without overloading the gallbladder with excessive fats.

Healthy Fats:

Choose healthy fats like those found in avocados, olive oil, and fatty fish. These support bile production and aid in the digestion of fats without straining the gallbladder.

Hydration: Stay adequately hydrated to maintain the flow of bile. Water is essential for overall digestive health and helps prevent the formation of gallstones.

Fiber Intake:

Include fiber-rich foods to regulate digestion and promote the regular movement of bile. Whole grains, fruits, and vegetables are excellent sources of dietary fiber.

Portion Control:

Practice mindful eating and control portion sizes. Avoid overeating, which can stress the gallbladder and hinder its efficient functioning.

Avoid Rapid Weight Loss:

If weight loss is a goal, aim for a gradual and steady approach. Sudden weight loss may increase the risk of gallstone formation.

Limit Processed Foods:

Reduce the consumption of processed and fried foods, as these can contribute to inflammation and may lead to gallbladder discomfort.

Regular Physical Activity: Engage in regular exercise to maintain a healthy weight and promote overall well-being.

Physical activity supports digestive processes and aids in weight management.

Listen to Your Body:

Pay attention to how your body responds to different foods. If you experience digestive discomfort, identify potential triggers and adjust your diet accordingly.

Consult Healthcare Professionals:

Seek guidance from healthcare professionals, especially if you have pre-existing gallbladder conditions or concerns. They can provide personalized advice based on your health status.

Benefits of Gall Bladder Health for Beginners

Prioritizing gallbladder health brings numerous benefits for beginners, positively impacting overall well-being and digestive harmony.

A well-maintained gallbladder contributes to optimal digestion and nutrient absorption, fostering a range of advantages.

Efficient Fat Digestion: A healthy gallbladder efficiently releases bile, aiding in the breakdown and digestion of fats.

This ensures that essential fatty acids are absorbed, supporting overall nutrient balance.

Prevention of Gallstones:

Following gallbladder health principles helps prevent the formation of gallstones, minimizing the risk of painful conditions like cholecystitis and potential complications requiring medical intervention.

Reduced Digestive Discomfort:

Proper gallbladder function minimizes digestive discomfort, including bloating, gas, and indigestion. Beginners can enjoy meals without the fear of post-meal discomfort.

Balanced Weight Management:

Maintaining gallbladder health is closely tied to balanced weight management. By adopting a healthy diet and lifestyle, beginners can support weight goals and reduce the risk of obesity-related gallbladder issues.

Enhanced Nutrient Absorption:

An optimally functioning gallbladder ensures the efficient absorption of essential nutrients, including fat-soluble vitamins (A, D, E, K), promoting overall nutritional wellness.

Improved Energy Levels:

A well-supported digestive system leads to improved energy levels. Proper nutrient absorption enables the body to utilize energy more effectively.

Prevention of Digestive Disorders:

Gallbladder health is linked to the prevention of various digestive disorders, such as gallbladder inflammation (cholecystitis) and bile duct issues, contributing to a healthier gastrointestinal system.

Support for Liver Function:

The gallbladder works in tandem with the liver. A healthy gallbladder supports liver function by ensuring the proper release of bile, aiding in detoxification processes.

Preventive Approach:

Adopting gallbladder-friendly habits early on serves as a preventive approach, reducing the likelihood of developing serious gallbladder conditions in the future.

Tips on Gall Bladder Health for Beginners

For beginners navigating the path to gallbladder health, adopting simple yet impactful tips can make a significant difference in promoting digestive well-being:

Hydration is Key:

Drink an ample amount of water daily to maintain bile flow and prevent the formation of gallstones. Staying hydrated supports overall digestive health.

Mindful Fat Intake:

Embrace healthy fats found in avocados, olive oil, and fatty fish while moderating saturated and trans fats. This supports optimal bile production and fat digestion.

Fiber-Rich Choices: Prioritize fiber-rich foods like fruits, vegetables, and whole grains. Fiber aids digestion and helps regulate the release of bile from the gallbladder.

Balanced Meals:

Plan balanced meals that include a mix of lean proteins, healthy fats, and complex carbohydrates. This ensures a steady and controlled release of bile during digestion.

Portion Control:

Practice portion control to prevent overeating. Smaller, well-distributed meals throughout the day reduce stress on the gallbladder.

Avoid Rapid Weight Loss:

If weight loss is a goal, pursue gradual and sustainable methods. Sudden weight loss can increase the risk of gallstone formation.

Limit Processed Foods:

Minimize the intake of processed and fried foods, as they can contribute to inflammation and gallbladder strain.

Regular Physical Activity:

Engage in regular exercise to support overall digestive health and weight management. Physical activity stimulates bile release and aids in maintaining a healthy weight.

Include Herbal Support:

Certain herbs like peppermint and turmeric may offer support for gallbladder health. Consult with healthcare professionals before incorporating herbal supplements.

Listen to Your Body:

Pay attention to how your body responds to different foods. Identify and avoid triggers that may cause discomfort or digestive distress.

Guidelines for Gall Bladder Health for Beginners

Embarking on a journey to maintain gallbladder health as a beginner involves embracing practical guidelines that foster digestive balance and overall well-being:

Nutrient-Rich Diet: Prioritize a nutrient-rich diet with a diverse range of fruits, vegetables, lean proteins, and whole grains. This ensures a well-rounded intake of essential vitamins and minerals.

Moderate Fat Consumption:

Embrace healthy fats like those found in avocados, nuts, and olive oil while limiting saturated and trans fats. Moderation in fat consumption supports optimal gallbladder function.

Regular Meal Timing: Establish regular meal timings to promote a consistent release of bile. Avoid prolonged periods between meals to prevent gallbladder stasis.

Hydration Habits:

Stay adequately hydrated by drinking water throughout the day. Hydration supports bile flow, preventing the formation of gallstones.

Fiber Inclusion:

Integrate fiber-rich foods into your diet to regulate digestion and support the gallbladder in releasing bile when needed.

Mindful Eating: Practice mindful eating by savoring each bite and paying attention to hunger and fullness cues. This helps prevent overeating and supports gallbladder health.

Regular Physical Activity:

Engage in regular physical activity to support overall digestive health and maintain a healthy weight. Exercise stimulates bile production and promotes efficient digestion.

Limit Processed Foods:

Minimize the consumption of processed and fried foods, which can contribute to inflammation and strain on the gallbladder.

Avoid Rapid Weight Loss: If weight loss is a goal, pursue gradual and sustainable methods to prevent the formation of gallstones associated with rapid weight loss.

Consult Healthcare Professionals:

Seek guidance from healthcare professionals for personalized advice, especially if you have existing gallbladder conditions or concerns. They can provide tailored recommendations based on your health status.

Adhering to these guidelines creates a foundation for gallbladder health, empowering beginners to make informed choices that contribute to digestive harmony and overall wellness.

Consistency in following these principles ensures a proactive approach to gallbladder health, fostering a resilient and balanced digestive system.

CHAPTER TWO

Healthy GallBladder Recipes for Beginners

1. Avocado and Chickpea Salad Bowl

Ingredients:

> - 1 can chickpeas, drained and rinsed
> - 1 avocado, diced
> - Cherry tomatoes, halved
> - Cucumber, diced
> - Olive oil and lemon dressing
> - Fresh cilantro for garnish

Instructions:

> - Combine chickpeas, avocado, tomatoes, and cucumber.
> - Drizzle with olive oil and lemon dressing.
> - Garnish with fresh cilantro.

Health Benefits:

> - Chickpeas provide fiber and protein.
> - Avocado offers healthy fats.

Preparation Time: 15 minutes

2. Quinoa and Vegetable Stir-Fry

Ingredients:

- ➤ 1 cup cooked quinoa
- ➤ Mixed vegetables (bell peppers, broccoli, carrots)
- ➤ 2 tablespoons coconut aminos
- ➤ 1 tablespoon olive oil
- ➤ Herbs and spices for seasoning

Instructions:

- ➤ Sauté mixed vegetables in olive oil.
- ➤ Add cooked quinoa and coconut aminos.
- ➤ Season with herbs and spices.

Health Benefits:

- ➤ Quinoa provides protein and fiber.
- ➤ Vegetables offer essential nutrients.

Preparation Time: 20 minutes

3. Salmon and Asparagus Foil Packets

Ingredients:

- ➤ 2 salmon fillets

- ➢ Asparagus spears
- ➢ Lemon slices
- ➢ Garlic, minced
- ➢ Olive oil
- ➢ Salt and pepper to taste

Instructions:

- ➢ Preheat the oven to 375°F (190°C).
- ➢ Place salmon on foil, surround with asparagus.
- ➢ Drizzle with olive oil, add garlic, lemon slices, salt, and pepper.
- ➢ Seal the foil and bake for 20 minutes.

Health Benefits:

- ➢ Salmon provides omega-3 fatty acids.
- ➢ Asparagus is a natural diuretic.

Preparation Time: 25 minutes

4. Turmeric and Ginger Carrot Soup

Ingredients:

- ➢ 4 cups carrots, chopped
- ➢ 1 onion, diced

- ➤ 2 teaspoons turmeric powder
- ➤ 1 teaspoon ginger, grated
- ➤ Vegetable broth
- ➤ Coconut milk (optional)

Instructions:

- ➤ Sauté onion, add carrots, turmeric, and ginger.
- ➤ Pour in vegetable broth, simmer until carrots are tender.
- ➤ Blend until smooth. Add coconut milk if desired.

Health Benefits:

- ➤ Turmeric and ginger have anti-inflammatory properties.
- ➤ Carrots provide vitamins.

Preparation Time: 30 minutes

5. Chicken and Broccoli Stir-Fry

Ingredients:

- ➤ 2 chicken breasts, sliced
- ➤ Broccoli florets
- ➤ 2 tablespoons coconut aminos
- ➤ Garlic, minced

- ➢ 1 tablespoon sesame oil
- ➢ Sesame seeds for garnish

Instructions:

- ➢ Cook sliced chicken in sesame oil until browned.
- ➢ Add broccoli and garlic, stir-fry until tender.
- ➢ Season with coconut aminos, garnish with sesame seeds.

Health Benefits:

- ➢ Chicken offers lean protein.
- ➢ Broccoli is rich in antioxidants.

Preparation Time: 25 minutes

6. Zucchini Noodles with Pesto

Ingredients:

- ➢ Zucchini noodles (zoodles)
- ➢ Cherry tomatoes, halved
- ➢ Pesto sauce (basil, pine nuts, olive oil)
- ➢ Parmesan cheese (optional)

Instructions:

- ➢ Spiralize zucchini into noodles.

- ➢ Toss with cherry tomatoes and pesto sauce.
- ➢ Top with Parmesan cheese if desired.

Health Benefits:

- ➢ Zoodles are low in carbs.
- ➢ Pesto provides healthy fats.

Preparation Time: 15 minutes

7. Baked Turkey and Sweet Potato Hash

Ingredients:

- ➢ 1 lb ground turkey
- ➢ Sweet potatoes, diced
- ➢ Onion, diced
- ➢ Bell peppers, chopped
- ➢ Smoked paprika, cumin, salt, and pepper

Instructions:

- ➢ Brown ground turkey, add diced sweet potatoes, onion, and bell peppers.
- ➢ Season with smoked paprika, cumin, salt, and pepper.
- ➢ Bake until sweet potatoes are tender.

Health Benefits:

- ➤ Turkey provides lean protein.
- ➤ Sweet potatoes offer vitamins and fiber.

Preparation Time: 35 minutes

8. Cauliflower Rice and Shrimp Bowl

Ingredients:

- ➤ Cauliflower rice
- ➤ Shrimp, peeled and deveined
- ➤ Garlic, minced
- ➤ Lemon juice
- ➤ Fresh parsley, chopped
- ➤ Olive oil

Instructions:

- ➤ Sauté shrimp in olive oil with garlic.
- ➤ Stir in cauliflower rice until cooked.
- ➤ Drizzle with lemon juice, garnish with parsley.

Health Benefits:

- ➤ Shrimp provides protein.
- ➤ Cauliflower rice is a low-carb alternative.

Preparation Time: 20 minutes

9. Lemon Herb Baked Cod

Ingredients:

- ➢ 4 cod fillets
- ➢ 2 tablespoons olive oil
- ➢ Lemon zest and juice
- ➢ Fresh herbs (dill, parsley)
- ➢ Garlic powder and onion powder
- ➢ Salt and pepper to taste

Instructions:

- ➢ Preheat the oven to 400°F (200°C).
- ➢ Place cod fillets on a baking sheet.
- ➢ Mix olive oil, lemon zest, lemon juice, herbs, and spices.
- ➢ Brush the mixture over cod fillets.
- ➢ Bake for 15-20 minutes until fish flakes easily.

Health Benefits:

- ➢ Cod is a lean protein source.
- ➢ Lemon and herbs provide flavor without added sugars.

Preparation Time: 25 minutes

10. Eggplant and Tomato Caprese Salad

Ingredients:

- ➤ 1 large eggplant, sliced
- ➤ Cherry tomatoes, halved
- ➤ Fresh mozzarella, sliced
- ➤ Basil leaves
- ➤ Balsamic glaze
- ➤ Olive oil

Instructions:

- ➤ Roast eggplant slices until tender.
- ➤ Arrange with cherry tomatoes and mozzarella.
- ➤ Top with fresh basil, drizzle with balsamic glaze and olive oil.

Health Benefits:

- ➤ Eggplant is low in carbs.
- ➤ Tomatoes and basil offer antioxidants.

Preparation Time: 30 minutes

11. Spinach and Mushroom Stuffed Chicken Breast

Ingredients:

- Chicken breasts
- Spinach, chopped
- Mushrooms, sliced
- Garlic, minced
- Olive oil
- Salt, pepper, and paprika for seasoning

Instructions:

- Sauté mushrooms and spinach in olive oil with garlic.
- Cut a pocket in chicken breasts, stuff with the sautéed mixture.
- Season with salt, pepper, and paprika.
- Bake until chicken is cooked through.

Health Benefits:

- Chicken provides lean protein.
- Spinach and mushrooms offer vitamins.

Preparation Time: 30 minutes

12. Cabbage and Turkey Skillet

Ingredients:

- ➤ Ground turkey
- ➤ Cabbage, shredded
- ➤ Onion, diced
- ➤ Garlic, minced
- ➤ Tomato sauce
- ➤ Italian seasoning

Instructions:

- ➤ Brown ground turkey with onion and garlic.
- ➤ Add shredded cabbage and tomato sauce.
- ➤ Season with Italian seasoning.
- ➤ Simmer until cabbage is tender.

Health Benefits:

- ➤ Turkey offers lean protein.
- ➤ Cabbage is low in calories and high in nutrients.

Preparation Time: 25 minutes

13. Mango and Black Bean Salad

Ingredients:

- ➢ Black beans, drained and rinsed
- ➢ Mango, diced
- ➢ Red onion, finely chopped
- ➢ Cilantro, chopped
- ➢ Lime juice
- ➢ Salt and cumin for seasoning

Instructions:

- ➢ Mix black beans, mango, red onion, and cilantro.
- ➢ Drizzle with lime juice.
- ➢ Season with salt and cumin.

Health Benefits:

- ➢ Black beans provide protein and fiber.
- ➢ Mango adds natural sweetness and vitamins.

Preparation Time: 15 minutes

14. Broccoli and Feta Omelette

Ingredients:

- ➢ Eggs

- ➢ Broccoli florets, steamed
- ➢ Feta cheese, crumbled
- ➢ Olive oil
- ➢ Salt and pepper to taste

Instructions:

- ➢ Whisk eggs and pour into a heated skillet.
- ➢ Add steamed broccoli and crumbled feta.
- ➢ Cook until eggs are set.
- ➢ Season with salt and pepper.

Health Benefits:

- ➢ Eggs provide protein.
- ➢ Broccoli is rich in fiber and nutrients.

Preparation Time: 15 minutes

15. Cilantro Lime Shrimp Salad

Ingredients:

- ➢ Shrimp, peeled and deveined
- ➢ Mixed greens
- ➢ Avocado, sliced
- ➢ Cherry tomatoes, halved
- ➢ Cilantro lime dressing

Instructions:

- ➢ Sauté shrimp until cooked.
- ➢ Arrange mixed greens, avocado, and tomatoes.
- ➢ Top with cooked shrimp.
- ➢ Drizzle with cilantro lime dressing.

Health Benefits:

- ➢ Shrimp provides lean protein.
- ➢ Avocado offers healthy fats.

Preparation Time: 20 minutes

16. Sesame Ginger Tofu Stir-Fry

Ingredients:

- ➢ Extra-firm tofu, cubed
- ➢ Mixed stir-fry vegetables
- ➢ Soy sauce or tamari
- ➢ Sesame oil
- ➢ Ginger, minced
- ➢ Garlic, minced

Instructions:

- ➢ Sauté tofu until golden.

- ➢ Stir-fry vegetables with ginger and garlic.
- ➢ Toss tofu and veggies with soy sauce and sesame oil.

Health Benefits:

- ➢ Tofu provides plant-based protein.
- ➢ Vegetables offer vitamins and fiber.

Preparation Time: 25 minutes

17. Sweet Potato and Turkey Chili

Ingredients:

- ➢ Ground turkey
- ➢ Sweet potatoes, diced
- ➢ Black beans, drained and rinsed
- ➢ Diced tomatoes
- ➢ Chili powder, cumin, and paprika
- ➢ Vegetable broth

Instructions:

- ➢ Brown turkey, add sweet potatoes, beans, and tomatoes.
- ➢ Season with chili powder, cumin, and paprika.
- ➢ Pour in vegetable broth, simmer until sweet potatoes are tender.

Health Benefits:

- ➤ Turkey provides lean protein.
- ➤ Sweet potatoes offer vitamins and fiber.

Preparation Time: 30 minutes

18. Caprese Stuffed Portobello Mushrooms

Ingredients:

- ➤ Portobello mushrooms
- ➤ Fresh mozzarella, sliced
- ➤ Tomatoes, sliced
- ➤ Basil leaves
- ➤ Balsamic glaze
- ➤ Olive oil

Instructions:

- ➤ Clean mushrooms and remove stems.
- ➤ Fill with mozzarella, tomatoes, and basil.
- ➤ Drizzle with balsamic glaze and olive oil.
- ➤ Bake until mushrooms are tender.

Health Benefits:

- ➤ Portobello mushrooms are low in calories.

> Tomatoes and basil offer antioxidants.

Preparation Time: 25 minutes

19. Pumpkin and Turkey Soup

Ingredients:

> Ground turkey
> Pumpkin puree
> Carrots, diced
> Onion, diced
> Garlic, minced
> Chicken broth
> Sage and thyme for seasoning

Instructions:

> Brown turkey, add onions, carrots, and garlic.
> Stir in pumpkin puree and chicken broth.
> Season with sage and thyme.
> Simmer until vegetables are tender.

Health Benefits:

> Turkey provides lean protein.
> Pumpkin is rich in vitamins and fiber.

Preparation Time: 30 minutes

20. Ratatouille with Quinoa

Ingredients:

- ➤ Eggplant, zucchini, bell peppers, tomatoes (sliced)
- ➤ Garlic, minced
- ➤ Olive oil
- ➤ Quinoa, cooked
- ➤ Fresh herbs (thyme, rosemary)
- ➤ Salt and pepper to taste

Instructions:

- ➤ Layer sliced vegetables in a baking dish.
- ➤ Drizzle with olive oil and sprinkle with garlic.
- ➤ Roast until vegetables are tender.
- ➤ Serve over cooked quinoa, garnish with fresh herbs.

Health Benefits:

- ➤ Quinoa provides protein and fiber.
- ➤ Ratatouille vegetables offer antioxidants.

Preparation Time: 35 minutes

21. Lemon Garlic Herb Baked Chicken Thighs

Ingredients:

- ➢ Chicken thighs
- ➢ Lemon juice
- ➢ Garlic, minced
- ➢ Fresh herbs (rosemary, thyme)
- ➢ Olive oil
- ➢ Salt and pepper to taste

Instructions:

- ➢ Marinate chicken thighs in lemon juice, garlic, herbs, and olive oil.
- ➢ Bake until chicken is golden and cooked through.

Health Benefits:

- ➢ Chicken thighs provide flavorful protein.
- ➢ Lemon and herbs add antioxidants.

Preparation Time: 30 minutes

22. Cucumber and Dill Greek Salad

Ingredients:

- ➢ Cucumbers, sliced

- ➢ Cherry tomatoes, halved
- ➢ Red onion, thinly sliced
- ➢ Feta cheese, crumbled
- ➢ Kalamata olives
- ➢ Greek dressing

Instructions:

- ➢ Combine cucumbers, tomatoes, red onion, feta, and olives.
- ➢ Drizzle with Greek dressing and toss gently.

Health Benefits:

- ➢ Cucumbers are hydrating.
- ➢ Feta provides calcium and protein.

Preparation Time: 15 minutes

23. Butternut Squash and Turkey Skillet

Ingredients:

- ➢ Ground turkey
- ➢ Butternut squash, diced
- ➢ Onion, diced
- ➢ Sage, thyme, and nutmeg for seasoning
- ➢ Olive oil

Instructions:

- ➤ Brown turkey with onion in olive oil.
- ➤ Add diced butternut squash and seasonings.
- ➤ Sauté until squash is tender.

Health Benefits:

- ➤ Turkey offers lean protein.
- ➤ Butternut squash is rich in vitamins.

Preparation Time: 25 minutes

24. Mushroom and Spinach Stuffed Bell Peppers

Ingredients:

- ➤ Bell peppers, halved
- ➤ Mushrooms, chopped
- ➤ Spinach, chopped
- ➤ Quinoa, cooked
- ➤ Mozzarella cheese
- ➤ Marinara sauce

Instructions:

- ➤ Sauté mushrooms and spinach.

- ➢ Mix with cooked quinoa.
- ➢ Stuff bell peppers, top with mozzarella.
- ➢ Bake until peppers are tender.

Health Benefits:

- ➢ Spinach provides iron and vitamins.
- ➢ Quinoa offers protein and fiber.

Preparation Time: 30 minutes

25. Cauliflower and Broccoli Gratin

Ingredients:

- ➢ Cauliflower and broccoli florets
- ➢ Garlic, minced
- ➢ Gruyere cheese, grated
- ➢ Parmesan cheese
- ➢ Milk or unsweetened almond milk
- ➢ Dijon mustard

Instructions:

- ➢ Steam cauliflower and broccoli until tender.
- ➢ Mix with minced garlic and transfer to a baking dish.
- ➢ Whisk milk, Dijon mustard, and grated cheeses.
- ➢ Pour over vegetables and bake until golden.

Health Benefits:

> ➤ Cauliflower and broccoli offer fiber and vitamins.
> ➤ Cheeses provide calcium and flavor.

Preparation Time: 35 minutes

26. Chia Seed Pudding with Berries

Ingredients:

> ➤ Chia seeds
> ➤ Almond milk
> ➤ Vanilla extract
> ➤ Mixed berries
> ➤ Maple syrup (optional)

Instructions:

> ➤ Mix chia seeds, almond milk, and vanilla extract.
> ➤ Refrigerate overnight.
> ➤ Top with mixed berries and drizzle with maple syrup if desired.

Health Benefits:

> ➤ Chia seeds are rich in omega-3 fatty acids.
> ➤ Berries offer antioxidants and vitamins.

Preparation Time: Overnight + 10 minutes

27. Cabbage and Apple Slaw

Ingredients:

- ➤ Green cabbage, shredded
- ➤ Apples, thinly sliced
- ➤ Greek yogurt
- ➤ Apple cider vinegar
- ➤ Honey
- ➤ Poppy seeds

Instructions:

- ➤ Toss shredded cabbage and sliced apples.
- ➤ Mix Greek yogurt, apple cider vinegar, honey, and poppy seeds.
- ➤ Dress the slaw with the mixture.

Health Benefits:

- ➤ Cabbage is low in calories and high in nutrients.
- ➤ Apples provide fiber and natural sweetness.

Preparation Time: 15 minutes

28. Spaghetti Squash with Pesto and Cherry Tomatoes

Ingredients:

- ➢ Spaghetti squash, roasted and shredded
- ➢ Pesto sauce
- ➢ Cherry tomatoes, halved
- ➢ Pine nuts (optional)
- ➢ Parmesan cheese (optional)

Instructions:

- ➢ Roast spaghetti squash and shred the flesh.
- ➢ Toss with pesto sauce.
- ➢ Top with cherry tomatoes and optional pine nuts or Parmesan.

Health Benefits:

- ➢ Spaghetti squash is a low-carb alternative.
- ➢ Pesto provides healthy fats.

Preparation Time: 40 minutes

29. Miso-Glazed Salmon with Bok Choy

Ingredients:

- ➢ Salmon fillets
- ➢ Miso paste
- ➢ Soy sauce or tamari
- ➢ Ginger, grated
- ➢ Bok choy, halved
- ➢ Sesame seeds for garnish

Instructions:

- ➢ Mix miso paste, soy sauce, and grated ginger.
- ➢ Brush the mixture over salmon.
- ➢ Roast until salmon is cooked.
- ➢ Sauté bok choy until tender.
- ➢ Serve salmon over bok choy, garnish with sesame seeds.

Health Benefits:

- ➢ Salmon provides omega-3 fatty acids.
- ➢ Bok choy is rich in vitamins.

Preparation Time: 30 minutes

30. Blueberry Almond Overnight Oats

Ingredients:

- ➤ Rolled oats
- ➤ Almond milk
- ➤ Greek yogurt
- ➤ Blueberries
- ➤ Almond butter
- ➤ Honey (optional)

Instructions:

- ➤ Mix rolled oats, almond milk, and Greek yogurt.
- ➤ Refrigerate overnight.
- ➤ Top with blueberries, almond butter, and honey if desired.

Health Benefits:

- ➤ Oats offer fiber and sustained energy.
- ➤ Blueberries are rich in antioxidants.

Preparation Time: Overnight + 10 minutes

31. Lentil and Vegetable Soup

Ingredients:

- Lentils, rinsed
- Carrots, diced
- Celery, chopped
- Onion, diced
- Garlic, minced
- Vegetable broth
- Cumin, coriander, and turmeric for seasoning

Instructions:

- Sauté onion and garlic, add carrots and celery.
- Stir in lentils, vegetable broth, and seasonings.
- Simmer until lentils are tender.

Health Benefits:

- Lentils provide plant-based protein and fiber.
- Vegetables offer essential nutrients.

Preparation Time: 40 minutes

32. Stuffed Acorn Squash with Quinoa and Cranberries

Ingredients:

- ➢ Acorn squash, halved and seeds removed
- ➢ Quinoa, cooked
- ➢ Dried cranberries
- ➢ Pecans, chopped
- ➢ Maple syrup
- ➢ Cinnamon for seasoning

Instructions:

- ➢ Roast acorn squash until tender.
- ➢ Mix quinoa, cranberries, and pecans.
- ➢ Stuff the squash, drizzle with maple syrup, and sprinkle with cinnamon.

Health Benefits:

- ➢ Acorn squash is rich in vitamins.
- ➢ Quinoa provides protein and fiber.

Preparation Time: 45 minutes

33. Tuna and White Bean Salad

Ingredients:

> ➤ Canned tuna, drained
> ➤ White beans, drained and rinsed
> ➤ Cherry tomatoes, halved
> ➤ Red onion, finely chopped
> ➤ Olive oil and lemon dressing
> ➤ Fresh parsley for garnish

Instructions:

> ➤ Combine tuna, white beans, tomatoes, and red onion.
> ➤ Drizzle with olive oil and lemon dressing.
> ➤ Garnish with fresh parsley.

Health Benefits:

> ➤ Tuna provides protein and omega-3 fatty acids.
> ➤ White beans offer fiber and minerals.

Preparation Time: 20 minutes

34. Cinnamon Apple Quinoa Breakfast Bowl

Ingredients:

> ➤ Quinoa, cooked

- ➢ Apples, diced
- ➢ Cinnamon
- ➢ Almond butter
- ➢ Walnuts, chopped
- ➢ Maple syrup (optional)

Instructions:

- ➢ Mix cooked quinoa with diced apples and cinnamon.
- ➢ Top with almond butter and chopped walnuts.
- ➢ Drizzle with maple syrup if desired.

Health Benefits:

- ➢ Quinoa provides protein and fiber.
- ➢ Apples offer vitamins and natural sweetness.

Preparation Time: 15 minutes

35. Mediterranean Chickpea Salad

Ingredients:

- ➢ Canned chickpeas, drained and rinsed
- ➢ Cucumber, diced
- ➢ Cherry tomatoes, halved
- ➢ Red onion, finely chopped
- ➢ Feta cheese, crumbled

> Greek dressing

Instructions:

> Combine chickpeas, cucumber, tomatoes, onion, and feta.
> Drizzle with Greek dressing and toss gently.

Health Benefits:

> Chickpeas provide protein and fiber.
> Feta adds calcium and flavor.

Preparation Time: 15 minutes

36. Brussels Sprouts and Almond Stir-Fry

Ingredients:

> Brussels sprouts, halved
> Almonds, sliced
> Garlic, minced
> Olive oil
> Lemon zest
> Red pepper flakes (optional)

Instructions:

> Sauté Brussels sprouts in olive oil until golden.

- ➢ Add sliced almonds, minced garlic, and lemon zest.
- ➢ Toss until Brussels sprouts are tender.
- ➢ Sprinkle with red pepper flakes if desired.

Health Benefits:

- ➢ Brussels sprouts are rich in fiber and vitamins.
- ➢ Almonds provide healthy fats.

Preparation Time: 20 minutes

37. Shredded Carrot and Pineapple Salad

Ingredients:

- ➢ Shredded carrots
- ➢ Pineapple chunks
- ➢ Greek yogurt
- ➢ Honey
- ➢ Chia seeds (optional)

Instructions:

- ➢ Combine shredded carrots and pineapple chunks.
- ➢ Mix Greek yogurt and honey for the dressing.
- ➢ Drizzle over the salad and sprinkle with chia seeds.

Health Benefits:

- ➢ Carrots offer beta-carotene and fiber.
- ➢ Pineapple adds natural sweetness.

Preparation Time: 15 minutes

38. Cherry Tomato and Basil Frittata

Ingredients:

- ➢ Cherry tomatoes, halved
- ➢ Fresh basil, chopped
- ➢ Eggs
- ➢ Feta cheese, crumbled
- ➢ Salt and pepper to taste

Instructions:

- ➢ Preheat the oven to 375°F (190°C).
- ➢ Whisk eggs and season with salt and pepper.
- ➢ Pour eggs into a skillet, add tomatoes, basil, and feta.
- ➢ Bake until eggs are set.

Health Benefits:

- ➢ Eggs provide protein.
- ➢ Tomatoes and basil offer antioxidants.

Preparation Time: 25 minutes

39. Cabbage and Pineapple Coleslaw

Ingredients:

- Green cabbage, shredded
- Pineapple, diced
- Greek yogurt
- Dijon mustard
- Apple cider vinegar
- Celery seeds

Instructions:

- Mix shredded cabbage and diced pineapple.
- In a separate bowl, whisk Greek yogurt, Dijon mustard, vinegar, and celery seeds.
- Toss the coleslaw with the dressing.

Health Benefits:

- Cabbage is low in calories and high in nutrients.
- Pineapple adds natural sweetness and vitamins.

Preparation Time: 15 minutes

40. Mango and Shrimp Ceviche

Ingredients:

- ➤ Shrimp, cooked and diced
- ➤ Mango, diced
- ➤ Red onion, finely chopped
- ➤ Cilantro, chopped
- ➤ Lime juice
- ➤ Jalapeño, minced (optional)

Instructions:

- ➤ Combine shrimp, mango, red onion, and cilantro.
- ➤ Drizzle with lime juice and toss gently.
- ➤ Add minced jalapeño for extra spice if desired.

Health Benefits:

- ➤ Shrimp provides lean protein.
- ➤ Mango offers vitamins and natural sweetness.

Preparation Time: 20 minutes

CONCLUSION

Embracing a gallbladder-friendly lifestyle for beginners involves a harmonious combination of mindful dietary choices, hydration, and overall well-being practices.

By prioritizing nutrient-rich foods, moderate fat intake, and incorporating fiber into daily meals, individuals can support optimal gallbladder function and promote digestive health.

The principles of gallbladder health extend beyond the plate to include portion control, regular physical activity, and attentive listening to the body's signals.

Steering clear of processed foods, embracing gradual and sustainable weight management, and consulting healthcare professionals for personalized guidance contribute to a comprehensive approach.

From easy-to-follow recipes rich in lean proteins, healthy fats, and vibrant vegetables to simple yet effective tips for daily living, beginners can embark on a journey towards digestive balance.

Whether savoring a colorful salad or relishing a nourishing soup, each choice contributes to the overall well-being of the gallbladder.

In the pursuit of gallbladder health, the importance of individualized approaches cannot be overstated.

Every step taken, every meal enjoyed, and every healthy habit formed lays the foundation for sustained well-being.

Through these practices, beginners can empower themselves to foster gallbladder resilience, paving the way for a vibrant and digestive-healthy life.

Remember, small changes today lead to lasting benefits tomorrow, as the journey to gallbladder health is a steady and rewarding progression towards optimal vitality.